W9-BHJ-948

Jessica's X-Ray

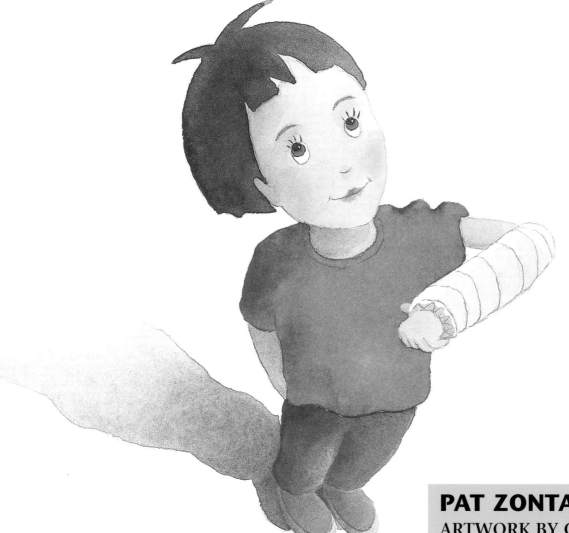

PAT ZONTA
ARTWORK BY CLIVE DOBSON

FIREFLY BOOKS

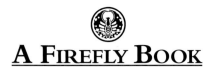

A FIREFLY BOOK

Published by Firefly Books Ltd., 2002

Second Printing, 2006

Library and Archives Canada Cataloguing in Publication

Zonta, Pat, 1951-
    Jessica's x-ray

Includes 6 x-rays printed on mylar.
ISBN-13: 978-1-55297-578-7 (bound)   ISBN-13: 978-1-55297-577-0 (pbk.)
ISBN-10: 1-55297-578-9 (bound)   ISBN-10: 1-55297-577-0 (pbk.)

    1. Radiography, Medical—Juvenile literature. 2. X-rays—Juvenile literature.
I. Dobson, Clive, 1949- II. Title.

RJ51.R3Z65 2002   j616.07'572   C2001-902624-2

Publisher Cataloging-in-Publication Data (U.S.)

Zonta., Pat.
    Jessica's x-ray / Pat Zonta ; artwork by Clive Dobson. — 1st ed.
[32] p. : ill. (some col.) : photos. ;   cm.
Summary: When Jessica goes to hospital after she breaks her arm, she learns about different x-ray techniques. Includes six actual x-ray images printed on film.
ISBN-13: 978-1-55297-578-7 (bound)   ISBN-13: 978-1-55297-577-0 (pbk.)
ISBN-10: 1-55297-578-9 (bound)   ISBN-10: 1-55297-577-0 (pbk.)

1. Radiology, Medical—Juvenile literature. I. Dobson, Clive. II. Title.
616.0757 21   CIP   2002

Published in Canada in 2002 by   Published in the United States in 2002 by
Firefly Books Ltd.   Firefly Books (U.S.) Inc.
66 Leek Crescent   P.O. Box 1338, Ellicott Station
Richmond Hill, Ontario L4B 1H1   Buffalo, New York 14205

The publisher gratefully acknowledges the financial support for our publishing program by the Canada Council for the Arts, the Ontario Arts Council and the Government of Canada through the Book Publishing Industry Development Program.

Printed in Singapore

For my family
In fulfillment of a promise

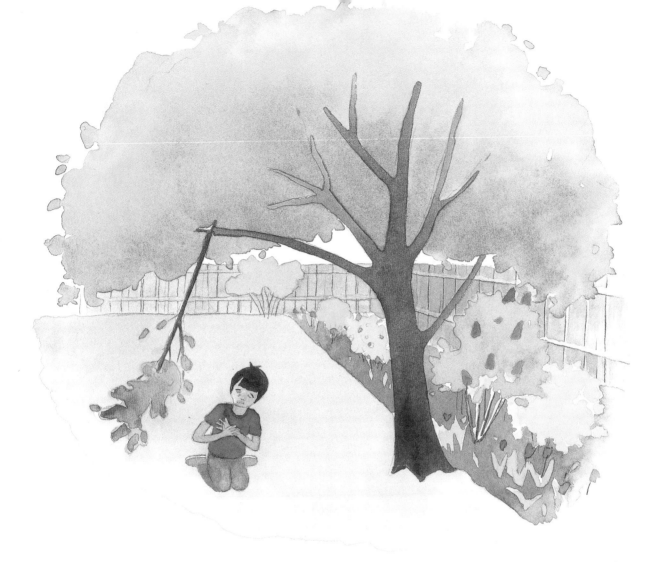

My name is Jessica. I was climbing a tree when I fell and broke my arm. Up to that point, my day had been perfect.

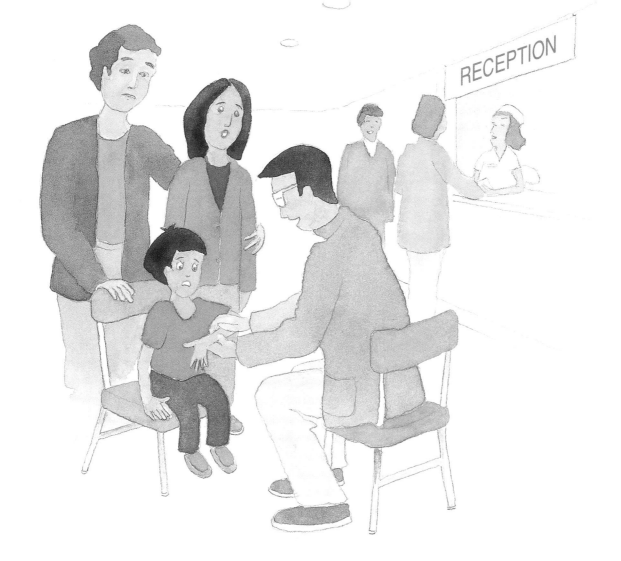

My parents took me to Children's Hospital where Doctor Dave looked at my arm. He said, "To help you get better as fast as possible, we need an x-ray to see what happened inside your arm."

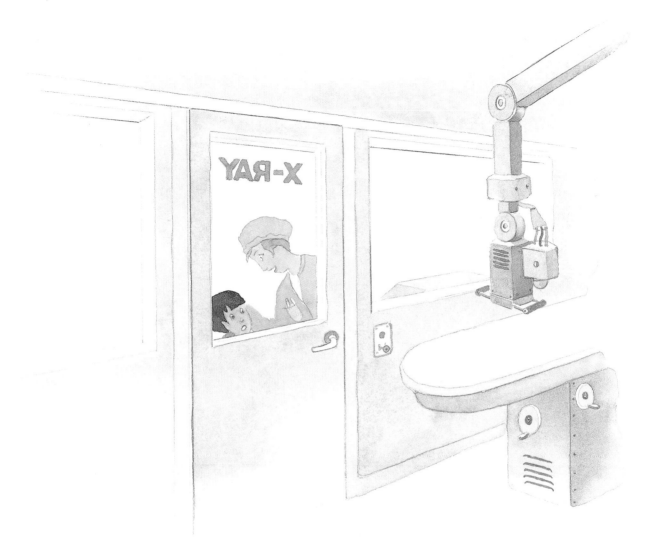

The x-ray room looked scary and I didn't want to go inside.
Sarah, the x-ray worker, said, "It's okay to be scared, Jessica,
but x-rays don't hurt. You can't feel or see them but they
zoom through your body and take pictures of your bones."

travel fast

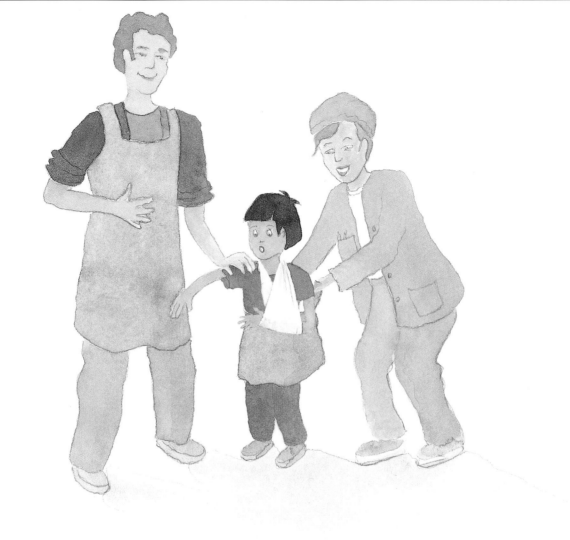

I felt better when Sarah let my Dad come in with me. "We only need to x-ray your arm," she said, "these lead aprons keep the x-rays away from other parts of your body."

This is an x-ray of a six-year-old child's hand. Can you count 26 bones? There are 27 bones in the hand and wrist of an adult (19 in the hand and 8 in the wrist).

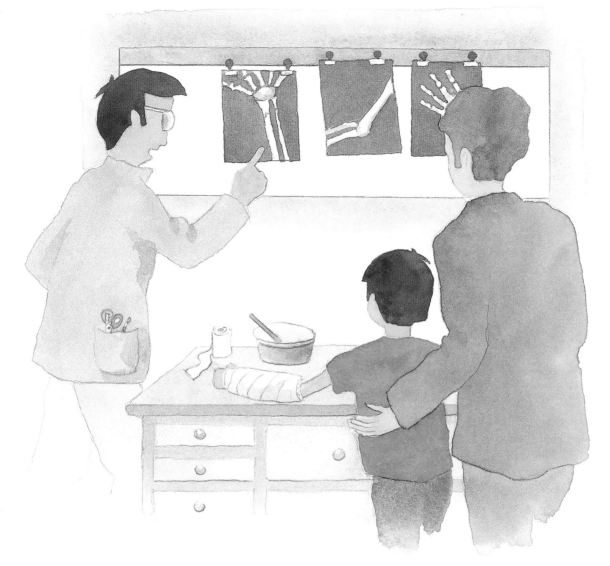

Sarah gave me three x-ray pictures to take to Doctor Dave.

He looked at them and said, "Your arm will get better soon.
I'll put a cast on now to help the bones heal properly. I'll check
the cast when it dries."

Did you know that the bones in your wrist grow in at different times as you grow up? Can you see where Jessica's arm is broken? Can you see where her bones are growing?

for help, please see page 28

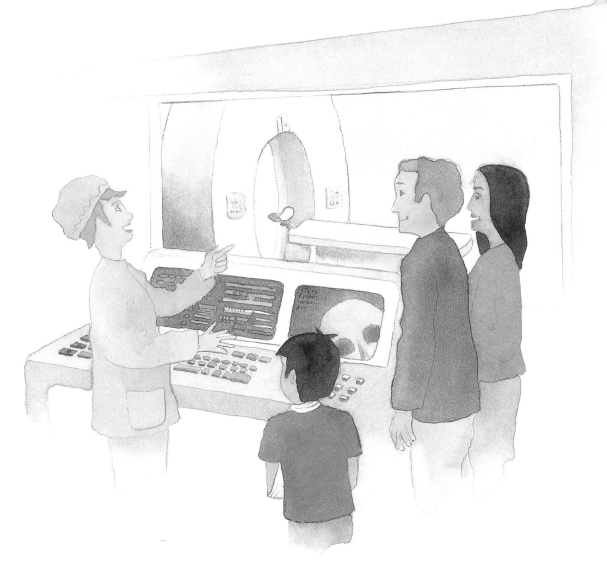

While we waited for my cast to dry, Sarah took us on a tour. We looked at a special x-ray called a CAT-scan which uses a computer to show things an ordinary x-ray can't see. The CAT-scan showed that a boy who had fallen off his bike was okay because he was wearing his helmet.

Your skull is made up of bones that fit together like a jigsaw puzzle to protect your brain. Can you see the skull? the brain? the scalp?

for help, please see page 28

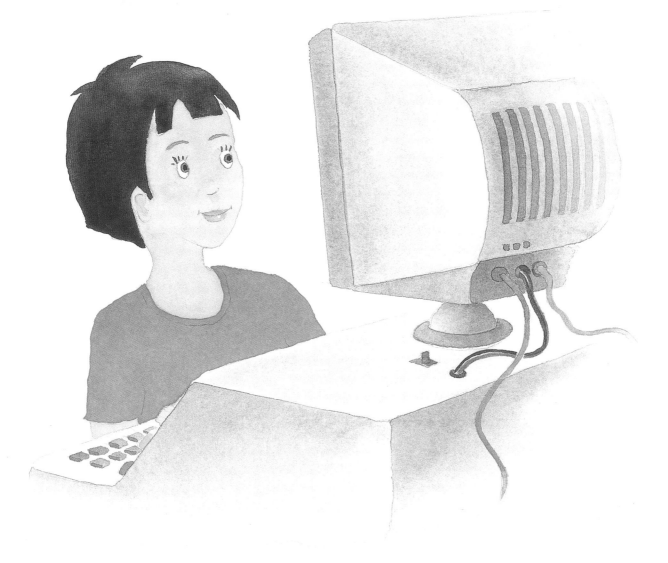

Sometimes babies swallow things they shouldn't. We saw an x-ray on a computer of a one-year-old boy who swallowed a penny. Doctors need an x-ray to show where the coin is to make sure it doesn't get stuck anywhere until it shows up in his diaper. "Yuck," I thought.

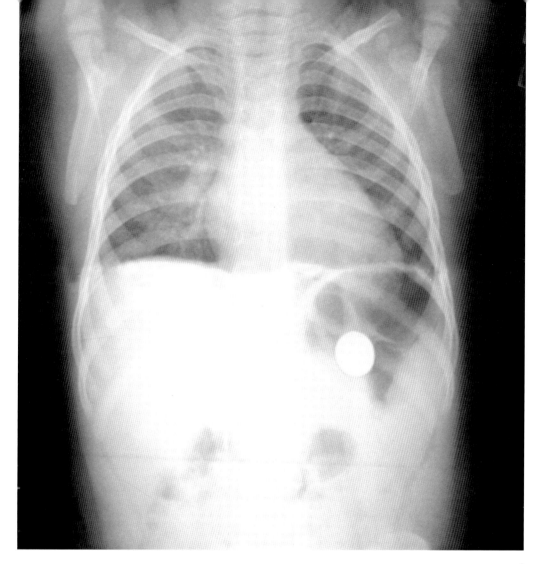

Healthy lungs look black on an x-ray. Can you see the coin? the
heart? the ribs? the collar bone?

for help, please see page 28

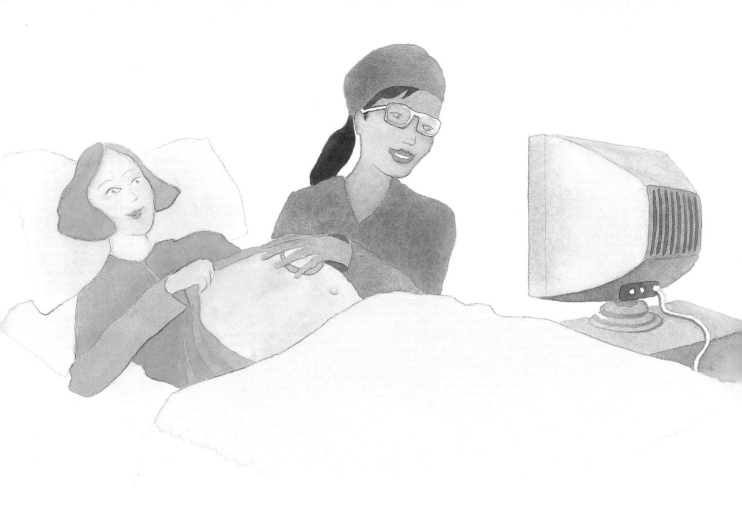

Not everyone who comes to a hospital is sick. Pregnant moms have an ultrasound to make sure the baby is okay.

Sarah said, "High-speed sound waves take a picture of the baby and can sometimes show if it is a boy or girl before it is born."

Mom said, "Jessica, on your ultrasound, you are sucking your thumb."

Can you see the baby? the head? the thumb? the spine?

for help, please see page 28

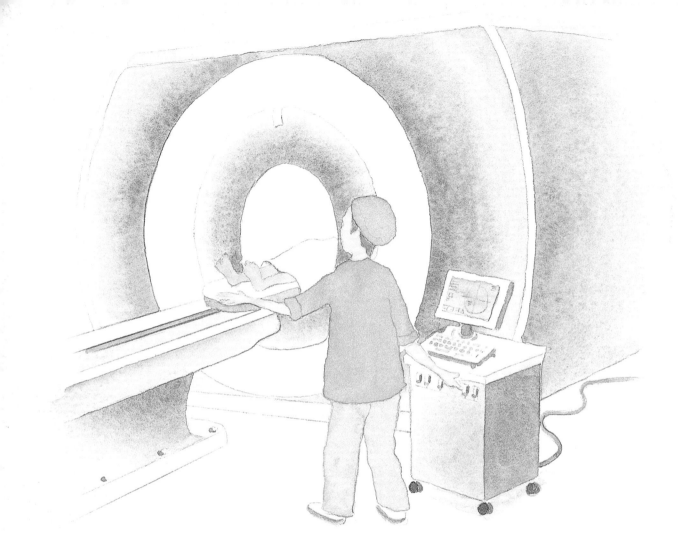

"Remember the CAT-scan picture of the boy's head?" Sarah asked. "There is another way we can see your brain. It's called an MRI machine and it uses a big magnet instead of x-rays to take pictures. The magnet is so strong it can pull the buckle right off your belt."

This is an MRI of a head. An MRI is used to show tissue that, in an ordinary x-ray, would be hidden behind the bone. Can you see the brain? the eyeballs? the pupils? the nose?

for help, please see page 28

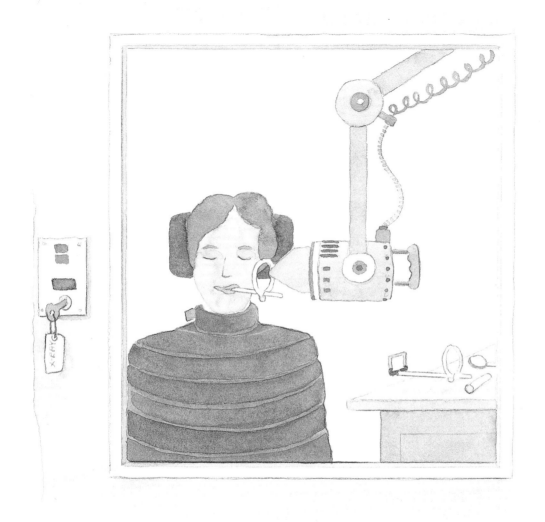

"This is where we take x-rays of your mouth," said Sarah.

We looked at an x-ray of a two-year-old. We could see his baby teeth and the molars that had not yet come through the gums.

Like bones, teeth are made of calcium and that's why we can see them on an x-ray. Can you see his ears? eye sockets? Can you see his baby teeth? Can you find where his molars are hiding?

for help, please see page 28

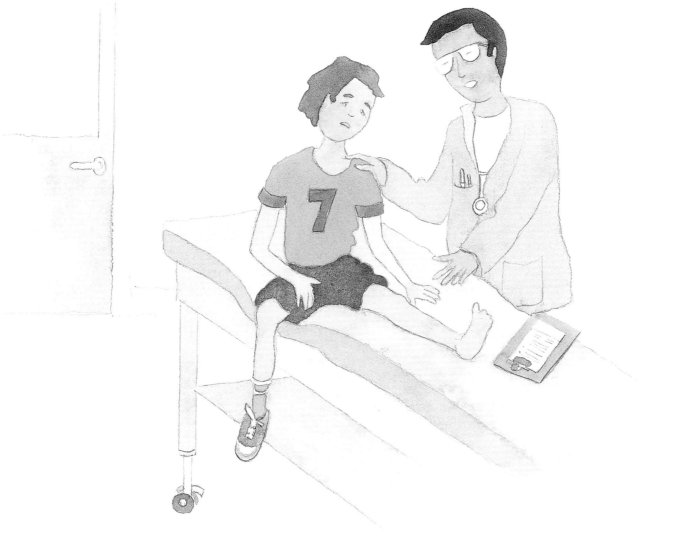

When we finished our tour, my cast was dry. We found Doctor Dave taking care of a boy with a broken leg in the emergency room.

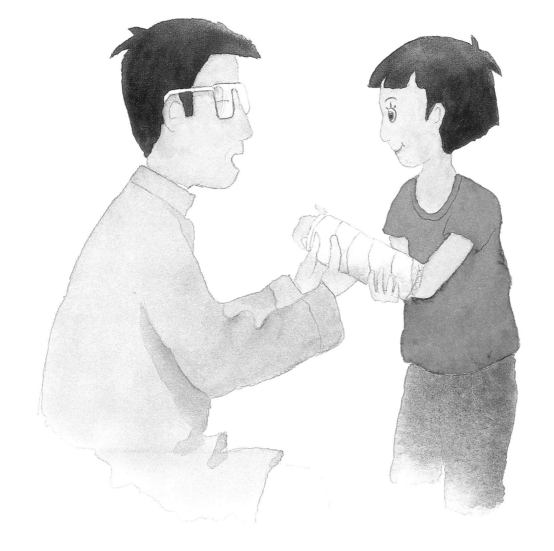

While he was waiting for the boy's x-rays, Doctor Dave checked my cast. He said, "Looks good, Jessica. We'll see you in a couple of weeks for a checkup. You have been a very brave girl."

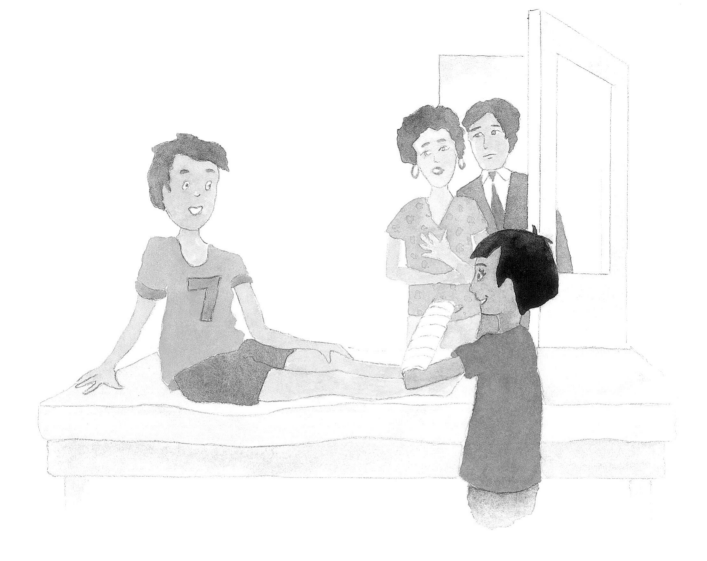

I thought the boy with the broken leg was brave too. His parents weren't at the hospital yet. He looked scared so I let him be the first to sign my cast. Then his parents ran through the door, just in time to see his first x-rays.

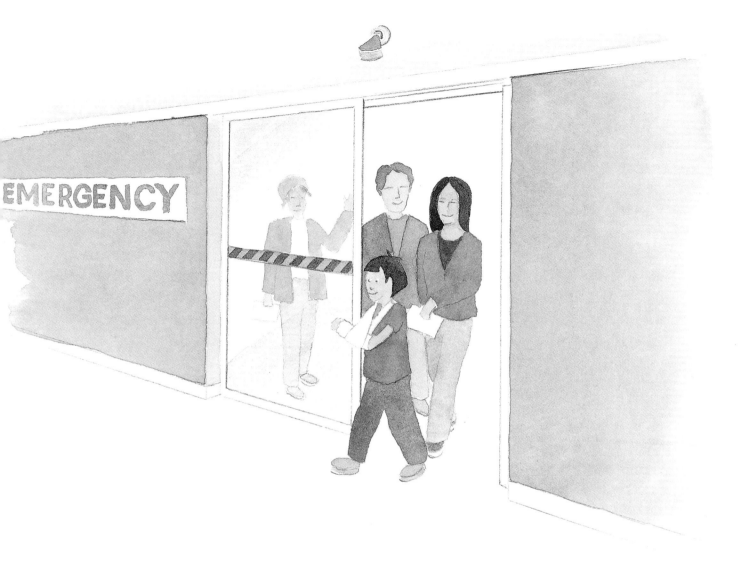

It had been an exciting day. I got to see inside a lot of people and I had a brand new cast for my friends to sign.

QUESTIONS AND ANSWERS ABOUT X-RAYS

Q. *What are x-rays?*

A. X-rays are invisible waves of energy that travel at the speed of light. An x-ray machine is similar to a camera but instead of light, it uses x-rays to make a picture. X-rays can't pass through the hard parts of your body (like bones and teeth) as easily as they can pass through the soft tissues (like skin, organs, and muscles). When x-rays go through your body they can create a picture on a computer screen or film. The hard parts show up lighter and the soft tissues show up as darker shades of gray.

Q. *How were x-rays discovered?*

A. X-rays were accidentally discovered by the German scientist William Roentgen while doing an experiment over 100 years ago. At first he didn't know what they were so he called them "x-rays" ("x" was short for "unknown").

Q. *Why do we have to wear a lead vest when we go into an x-ray room?*

A. X-rays are safe and helpful tools when they are used carefully by x-ray workers. X-rays can't pass through lead, so wearing a lead apron or vest stops x-rays from going through your body when your head, neck, arms, or legs are being x-rayed.

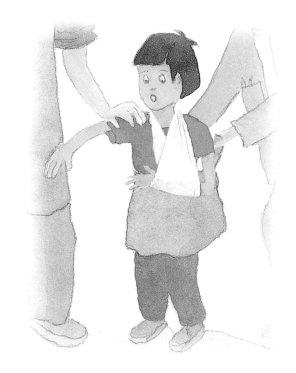

Q. *How do doctors decide if you need an x-ray?*

A. Doctors ask you to have an x-ray when they want to see the bones inside your body. If the doctor thinks your bone may be broken, an x-ray can show what your bone actually looks like.

Q. *When do doctors decide they need to send you for a CAT-scan?*

A. CAT-scans use x-rays. The letters CAT stand for "computed axial tomography." Doctors might ask for a CAT-scan (or CT as it is sometimes called) after an accident to see if there is any brain injury or cracks in the skull which an ordinary x-ray cannot show. An ordinary x-ray cannot show fine details about the condition of your organs, the tissues around your bones, or how blood is flowing through your brain, chest, or belly, but a CT can.

Q. *When do doctors decide they need to send you for an MRI?*

A. The letters MRI stand for "magnetic resonance imaging." Doctors might ask for an MRI when they want to see how your brain, spine and muscles are working. They will ask for an MRI when ordinary x-rays and CAT-scans cannot show if there is a problem in these places. An MRI doesn't use x-rays but uses magnetic waves.

Q. *Why do doctors ask for an ultrasound?*

A. Doctors might ask for an ultrasound to look for illness or bruising in the belly after an accident. Doctors also ask for an ultrasound when they are looking at a baby still in the mother's belly and when they need to check on the condition of organs in the body. An ultrasound uses sound waves that bounce from the imager through your body and back to the imager. An ultrasound is very safe.

SOLUTIONS

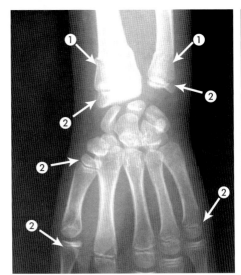

1. her arm is broken in two places
2. places where her bones are growing

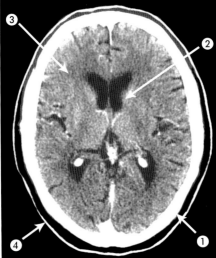

1. skull
2. ventricle (sacs filled with spinal fluid)
3. brain
4. scalp (skin)

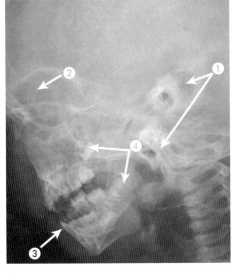

1. coin
2. heart
3. ribs
4. collar bone

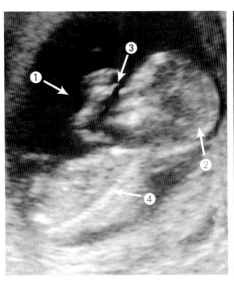

1. baby
2. head
3. thumb
4. spine

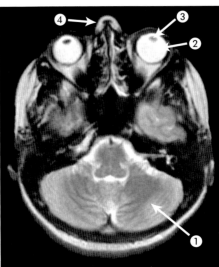

1. brain
2. eyeballs
3. pupils
4. nose

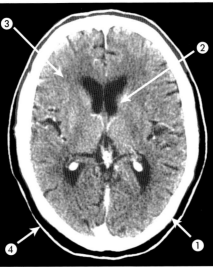

1. ears
2. eye sockets
3. baby teeth
4. molars